46 Meal Recipes to Increase Your Breast Milk Production:

Using the Best Natural Ingredients to Help Your Body Produce Healthy Milk for Your Baby

By

Joe Correa CSN

COPYRIGHT

ACKNOWLEDGEMENTS

This book is dedicated to my friends and family that have had mild or serious illnesses so that you may find a solution and make the necessary changes in your life.

46 Meal Recipes to Increase Your Breast Milk Production:

Using the Best Natural Ingredients to Help Your Body Produce Healthy Milk for Your Baby

By

Joe Correa CSN

CONTENTS

ABOUT THE AUTHOR

After years of Research, I honestly believe in the positive effects that proper nutrition can have over the body and mind. My knowledge and experience has helped me live healthier throughout the years and which I have shared with family and friends. The more you know about eating and drinking healthier, the sooner you will want to change your life and eating habits.

Nutrition is a key part in the process of being healthy and living longer so get started today. The first step is the most important and the most significant.

INTRODUCTION

46 Meal Recipes to Increase Your Breast Milk Production: Using the Best Natural Ingredients to Help Your Body Produce Healthy Milk for Your Baby

By Joe Correa CSN

The joyful closeness with your newborn baby through breastfeeding is definitely one of the most amazing experiences in life. A newborn baby, its growth and development progress, completely depends on the mother and the quality of her milk. A healthy mother means nutritious breastmilk which will give the baby strength in the first stage of life. When you choose to breastfeed, you're investing in your baby's future health.

Your body is a fantastic organism. It goes through millions of chemical processes each and every day to create the right balance of nutrients to help your newborn grow into a strong child. New mothers are often afraid to change their nutritional habits as that could affect their milk production. The lack of information during pregnancy leads to wrong conclusions.

In order to achieve the best results and provide your child with the essential nutrients for its development, you must put in the necessary effort. Eating the right amounts and types of food can help your child get the most out of breastfeeding.

Food amounts depend from one person to another depending on each individual's body. What you have to learn is to listen to your body's needs.

The short-term unbalanced diet during breastfeeding will not significantly affect breastmilk production. However, if you have some bad habits throughout a longer period of time, it will definitely have some undesirable effects on the quality and the quantity of your breastmilk and your baby's development in its most important stage.

Having this in mind, I have created these amazingly delicious recipes that will provide all the necessary nutrients you and your child need. I truly hope this book will make some positive changes in your life and give you some new and exciting meal ideas for every day of this wonderful journey you're about to take. I wanted to keep these recipes as simple as possible because I know how important every second with your precious one is.

Try every one of these recipes and enjoy this period of life. You deserve it!

46 MEAL RECIPES TO INCREASE YOUR BREAST MILK PRODUCTION: USING THE BEST NATURAL INGREDIENTS TO HELP YOUR BODY PRODUCE HEALTHY MILK FOR YOUR BABY

1.   Brussel Sprout Risotto

Ingredients:

1 lb lamb, tender cuts

1 cup rice

12 oz brussels sprouts

¼ cup sweet corn

4-5 pieces baby corn

2 tbsp butter, softened

1 tbsp turmeric, ground

1 tsp sea salt

¼ tsp freshly ground black pepper

3 cups lamb's broth

Preparation:

Rinse the meat under cold running water and pat dry with a kitchen paper. Place on a clean working surface and using a sharp knife, cut into bite-sized pieces. Place the meat at the bottom of a large, heavy-bottomed pot. Add three cups of water and cover with a lid. Simmer for 30 minutes, over medium heat.

Remove the meat but reserve the liquid for the rice. Now add rice and season with salt, pepper, and ground turmeric. Cook for another 8 minutes, stirring occasionally. Finally, add meat chops and give it a good stir. Cook for five more minutes.

Meanwhile, melt the butter in a large skillet. Add Brussels sprouts, corn, and baby corn. Cook for about 15 minutes, stirring constantly until the sprouts are nicely browned and lightly charred. Serve with rice and meat. Optionally, add some more pepper or salt to taste.

Nutrition information per serving: Kcal: 491, Protein: 34.8g, Carbs: 61.4g, Fats: 13.4g

2. Chicken Pudding with Artichoke

Ingredients:

1 lb dark and white chicken meat, cooked

2 artichokes

2 tbsp of butter, unsalted

2 tbsp of extra virgin olive oil

1 lemon, juiced

1 handful of fresh parsley leaves

1 tsp of pink Himalayan salt

¼ tsp of freshly ground black pepper

½ tsp of ground chili pepper, for topping

Preparation:

If possible, use organic chicken meat (breast and thighs). Thoroughly rinse the meat and pat dry with a kitchen paper. Using a sharp paring knife, cut the meat into smaller pieces and remove the bones. Rub with olive oil and set aside.

Heat the saute pan over medium-high heat. Turn the heat down slightly to medium and add the meat. Cook for about one minute to get it a little golden one one side. Then flip each piece, cover the pan with a thigh fitting lid and turn the heat to low. Cook for ten minutes without removing the lid. This will poach your meat from the inside out in its own juices. This is why it's important that the lid stays on all the time.

Now turn off the heat and let it sit for another ten minutes. It has to stay covered the whole time. Take the lid off the pan and set aside allowing the meat to cool for a while.

Meanwhile, prepare the artichoke. Cut the lemon into halves and squeeze the juice in a small bowl. Divide the juice in half and set aside.

Using a sharp paring knife, trim off the outer leaves until you reach the yellow and soft ones. Trim off the green outer skin around the artichoke base and stem. Make sure to remove the 'hairs' around the artichoke heart. They are inedible so simply throw them away. Cut artichoke into half-inch pieces. Rub with half of the lemon juice and place in a heavy-bottomed pot. Add enough water to cover and cook until completely fork-tender. Remove from the heat and drain. Chill for a while (to a room temperature). I like to cut each piece into thin strips, but this is optional.

Now combine artichoke with chicken meat in a large bowl. Stir in salt, pepper, and the remaining lemon juice. Melt the butter over medium heat and drizzle over pudding. Sprinkle with some chili pepper and parsley. Serve.

Nutrition information per serving: Kcal: 486, Protein: 47.4g, Carbs: 11.5g, Fats: 28.4g

3.   Chicken Risotto with Soaked Pide

Ingredients:

1 lb chicken meat, dark and white parts

½ cup rice

4 cups chicken broth

1 large pide bread, chopped into bite-sized pieces

1 tsp salt

½ tsp freshly ground black pepper

Sour cream for topping (optionally)

Preparation:

If possible, use organic chicken meat (breast and thighs). Thoroughly rinse the meat and pat dry with a kitchen paper. Using a sharp paring knife, cut the meat into smaller pieces and remove the bones. Rub with salt and place in a deep pot. Add 4 cups of chicken broth and cook for 30 minutes.

When the meat is fork-tender, remove from the pot but keep the liquid. Add rice and cook for 10 minutes, stirring occasionally.

Meanwhile, cut the chicken meat into bite-sized pieces and place in a large bowl. Set aside.

In another bowl, cut pide bread into bite-sized pieces. Add rice and the remaining broth to soak the pide bread. Stir in chicken chops and let it stand for 15 more minutes. Sason with salt and pepper before serving.

Optionally top with sour cream.

Nutrition information per serving: Kcal: 445, Protein: 43.7g, Carbs: 48.1g, Fats: 6.8g

4.   Braised Spinach and Leeks

Ingredients:

12 oz fresh spinach

3 large leeks, sliced

2 red onions, sliced

2 garlic cloves, crushed

½ cup goat's cheese

3 tbsp extra virgin olive oil

1 tsp sea salt

Preparation:

Heat up the olive oil over medium-high heat. Add sliced leek, garlic, and onions. Stir-fry for about five minutes, over medium heat.

Now add spinach and give it a good stir. Season with sea salt and continue to cook for 3 more minutes, stirring constantly.

Remove from the heat and sprinkle with fresh goat's cheese.

Serve immediately.

Nutrition information per serving: Kcal: 301, Protein: 9.6g, Carbs: 24.7g, Fats: 20.4g

5.   Creamy Cheese Bread with Olive oil

Ingredients:

14 oz whole wheat flour

1 ¼ cup lukewarm water

2 tbsp olive oil

1 tsp baking powder

1 tsp honey

1 tsp salt

2 tbsp dry yeast

For filling:

1 cup Feta cheese

3 tbsp fresh rosemary, finely chopped

3 spring onions, sliced

2 garlic cloves, crushed

½ cup olives

6-7 peppercorns

¼ cup olive oil

Preparation:

Combine all dry ingredients in a large bowl. Gradually add water beating well after each addition. Now add olive oil and stir well. Cover with a clean towel and let it stand for 30 minutes at the room temperature.

Knead 10 to 15 minutes until dough is smooth and elastic. Place in a lightly greased bowl and let it rise for one hour.

Preheat the oven to 375 degrees and bake for 30 minutes. Remove from the oven chill for a while.

Using a sharp paring knife, cut the bread and fill with Feta cheese, finely chopped rosemary, crushed garlic, olives, peppercorns, and olive oil. Bake for 10 more minutes.

Remove from the oven and chill completely. Sprinkle with sliced spring onions and serve.

Nutrition information per serving: Kcal: 349, Protein: 8.1g, Carbs: 34.3g, Fats: 20.7g

6.   Mediterranean Scallops

Ingredients:

4 large Mediterranean scallops, cleaned

4 tbsp extra virgin olive oil

1 tsp sea salt

1 tsp garlic powder

1 tbsp freshly squeezed lemon juice

1 tsp dried rosemary

1 cup white wine

Preparation:

Rinse well scallops under cold running water. Place in a heavy-bottomed pot and pour in white wine, rosemary, lemon juice, garlic powder, salt, and olive oil. Add one cup of water and bring it to a boil. Cook until barely tender, 3-4 minutes. Reduce the heat to medium and simmer for ten more minutes.

Remove from the heat and chill for a while. Place each scallop on a serving plate and brush with the remaining liquid.

Serve with wild asparagus salad.

Nutrition information per serving: Kcal: 340, Protein: 20.9g, Total Carb: 9.2g, Dietary Fiber: 0.9g, Sugars: 1.9g, Total Fat: 15.2g, Saturated Fat: 2.3g

7.   Wild asparagus salad

Ingredients:

7 oz fresh wild asparagus

3 tbsp extra virgin olive oil

2 garlic cloves, crushed

2 tbsp freshly squeezed lemon juice

½ tsp sea salt

Preparation:

Rinse well the asparagus and cut into one-inch-long pieces. Drain and set aside.

Heat up the olive oil in a large non-stick skillet. Add garlic and stir-fry for three minutes. Now add asparagus and continue to cook for ten more minutes, stirring constantly.

Remove from the heat and season with salt and lemon juice.

8.   Spring Vegetable Soup

Ingredients:

1 medium-sized carrot, finely chopped

2 spring onions, finely chopped

1 yellow bell pepper, finely chopped and seeds removed

2 celery stalks, finely chopped

½ cup celery leaves, finely chopped

½ tsp dried thyme

2 tbsp butter

1 tsp vegetable oil

4 cups vegetable broth

1 cup milk

1 tsp salt

¼ tsp black pepper, freshly ground

Preparation:

Heat up the oil in a large, heavy-bottomed pan. Add butter and allow it to melt. Now add finely chopped carrot, spring onions, bell pepper, and celery stalks. Cook for ten minutes, stirring constantly.

Pour in vegetable broth and bring it to a boil. Reduce the heat to medium and add milk, celery leaves, thyme, salt, and pepper.

Cook for 15 minutes stirring occasionally.

Nutrition information per serving: Kcal: 150, Protein: 7.6g, Total Carb: 8.6g, Dietary Fiber: 1.2g, Sugars: 6g, Total Fat: 9.6g, Saturated Fat: 5g

9.　　Bell Pepper Risotto with Chicken

Ingredients:

12 oz of chicken breasts, boneless, skinless, and cut into bite-sized pieces

1 cup of rice

7 oz of button mushrooms, sliced

1 red bell pepper, halved and seeds removed

1 green bell pepper, halved and seeds removed

1 yellow bell pepper, halved and seeds removed

7 oz of cauliflower florets

5-6 baby corn

½ cup of sweet corn

2 medium-sized carrots, peeled and chopped

2 tbsp of olive oil

1 tbsp of butter

1 tsp of salt

½ tsp of freshly ground black pepper

1 tsp of fresh rosemary, finely chopped

Preparation:

First, you will have to prepare the rice. Place one cup of rice in a deep pot. Add 3 cups of water and a pinch of salt. Bring it to a boil and reduce the heat to medium-low. Cook until the water evaporates, stirring occasionally. Remove from the heat and set aside.

Rinse and clean the vegetables. Pat dry and cut each pepper in half. Remove the seeds and thinly slice, or chop each pepper. Finely chop the carrots because they take a long time to cook, so you want them as smaller as possible. Divide cauliflower into small florets. Remove the stems from button mushrooms and slice them.

Now, grease a large skillet with two tablespoons of oil and add carrots and cauliflower. Cook for 15 minutes. Now, add corn, baby corn, and bell peppers. Continue to cook for 5 minutes, stirring constantly. Finally, add mushrooms, give it a good stir and cook for 3-4 minutes. Remove from the heat and combine with rice. Set aside.

Meanwhile, prepare the chicken. Rinse well the meat under cold running water and pat dry using a kitchen paper. Place on a clean working surface. With a sharp paring knife, gently remove the skin and bones. Chop chicken breasts into bite-sized pieces. Place in a deep pot and cook until fork tender. Drain and combine with rice and vegetables. Serve warm and optionally top with Greek yogurt.

Nutrition information per serving: Kcal: 530, Protein: 30.8g, Carbs: 73g, Dietary Fibers: 8.2g, Sugars: 12g, Fats: 15.5g, Saturated Fats: 4.1g

10.   Soft Chicken with Spinach

Ingredients:

2 lbs organic chicken meat, dark and white meat

5 oz fresh spinach, torn

2 cups of chicken broth, homemade

2 tbsp butter, unsalted

2 tbsp olive oil

1 tsp sea salt

Preparation:

If possible, use organic chicken meat (breast and thighs). Thoroughly rinse the meat and pat dry with a kitchen paper. Using a sharp paring knife, cut the meat into smaller pieces.

Rinse well the spinach. Always look for organic vegetables. They can be a bit messier to clean but are definitely worth it. Chop and drain in a colander.

Grease a large heavy-bottomed pot with olive oil. Place the meat in it and pour in two cups of chicken broth. Add salt and cook for about one hour over medium temperature. When the meat is completely fork-tender, remove from the heat and drain in a large colander. You can reserve the liquid for a nice chicken soup.

Melt the butter in a large skillet, over medium-high heat. Add chopped spinach and stir-fry for 3-4 minutes, stirring constantly. Now add ¼ cup of water and continue to cook until the water evaporates.

Serve together and season with some more salt if needed. I like to add some freshly ground turmeric before serving, but this is completely optional.

Nutrition information per serving: Kcal: 484, Protein: 57.8g, Carbs: 7.2g, Fats: 24.7g

11.   Chickpea Stew with Onions

Ingredients:

1 lb chickpeas, soaked

3 large purple onions, peeled and sliced

2 large tomatoes, roughly chopped

3 oz parsley, chopped

2 cups vegetable broth

1 tbsp cayenne pepper

3 tbsp butter

2 tbsp olive oil

1 tsp salt

½ tsp freshly ground black pepper

Preparation:

Heat up the oil in a large skillet. Add onions and cook until translucent. Now add soaked chickpeas, chopped tomatoes, chopped parsley, and vegetable broth. Stir in cayenne pepper, salt, and freshly ground black pepper.

Reduce the heat to minimum and simmer for 45 minutes, stirring occasionally. Serve warm.

Nutrition information per serving: Kcal: 513, Protein: 21.8g, Carbs: 68.3g, Dietary Fibers: 19.4g, Sugars: 16g, Fats: 19.1g, Saturated Fats: 6g

12.   Thick Tomato Stew

Ingredients:

2 lbs pork stew meat

1 large eggplant, chopped into bite-sized pieces

4 large tomatoes, peeled and roughly chopped

4 tbsp sunflower oil

2 bay leaves

2 tbsp of tomato paste, homemade

1 tbsp of Cayenne pepper, ground

½ tsp of chili pepper, ground (optional)

½ tsp of salt

Preparation:

Rinse the pork and season with salt and pepper.

Grease the bottom of a large, heavy-bottomed pot with oil. Heat up the oil over medium heat and add pork. Brown the meat on all sides for about 15 minutes. Now add tomatoes and eggplants and continue to cook for five more minutes, stirring constantly.

Reduce the heat to minimum and add two cups of water. Stir in two tablespoons of homemade tomato paste, cayenne pepper, and optionally chili pepper. Add two bay leaves and some more salt to taste. Cover and cook for about 45 minutes, or until pork is completely tender.

Nutrition information per serving: Kcal: 408, Protein: 49.7g, Carbs: 11.1g, Fats: 18.1g

13.   Cold Okra Salad

Ingredients:

7 oz fresh okra, whole

7 oz bean sprouts, trimmed

½ cup green peas, pre-cooked

2 medium-sized carrots, sliced into strips

7 oz cherry tomatoes, whole

3.5 oz baby corn, whole

3 garlic cloves, crushed

3 tbsp extra virgin olive oil

¼ cup vegetable broth

½ tsp sea salt

1 tbsp fresh rosemary, finely chopped

Preparation:

Rinse the vegetables and drain in a large colander. Peel and slice carrots into thin strips. Place in a large non-stick skillet and cook for 8-10 minutes, stirring constantly. Remove from the heat and set aside.

Now heat up the olive oil and add garlic and rosemary. Stir-fry until translucent, for about 3-4 minutes. Now add vegetables, vegetable broth, and salt. Cook until the liquid evaporates.

Remove from the heat and serve warm.

Nutrition information per serving: Kcal: 235, Protein: 7.4g, Carbs: 32.3g, Dietary Fibers: 6.3g, Sugars: 7.3g, Fats: 10.2g, Saturated Fats: 1.5g

14.   Collard Greens with Shrimps

Ingredients:

1 lb collard greens, chopped

1 lb shrimps, whole

7 oz octopus, chopped into bite-sized pieces

1 large tomato, peeled and finely chopped

3 cups fish stock

4 tbsp extra virgin olive oil

3 garlic cloves

2 tbsp fresh parsley, finely chopped

1 tsp sea salt

Preparation:

Rinse well the greens and drain in a large colander. Place on a clean working surface and chop with a sharp knife. Set aside.

Now place shrimps and octopus in a large, deep pot. Add chopped tomato and fish stock. Cover with a lid and cook for 40 minutes, over medium-high heat, until octopus is fork-tender. Remove from the heat and drain.

Now, grease the bottom of your pot with olive oil and add garlic and parsley. Stir-fry until translucent, stirring constanty.

Finally, add chopped collard greens and simmer for 10 more minutes. Season with salt and give it a good stir. Remove from the heat and serve with shrimps and octopus.

Nutrition information per serving: Kcal: 368, Protein: 40.3g, Carbs: 10.9g, Dietary Fibers: 4g, Sugars: 0g, Fats: 18.9g, Saturated Fats: 3.1g

15.   Collard Greens with Veal

Ingredients:

1 lb of veal brisket, cut into half-inch thick pieces

2 lbs of collard greens, torn

¼ cup of rice

2 garlic cloves, crushed

¼ cup of olive oil

2 tsp of sea salt

½ lemon, juiced

Preparation:

Rinse well the meat under the running water. Pat dry using a kitchen paper and sprinkle with salt. Set aside.

Heat up three tablespoons of olive oil in a large pot. Add meat and briefly brown on all sides. Now add about one cup of water and reduce the heat. Simmer until fork tender. Now add rice and one more cup of water. Continue to cook until the liquid evaporates.

Add greens, garlic, and the remaining olive oil. Cover with a lid and simmer for five minutes over minimum temperature.

Serve warm.

Nutrition information per serving: Kcal: 410, Protein: 33.5g, Carbs: 22.2g, Dietary Fibers: 7.7g, Sugars: 0g, Fats: 22.8g, Saturated Fats: 5.3g

16.   Fresh Tomato and Celery Soup

Ingredients:

1 lb tomatoes, peeled and roughly chopped

3.5 oz celery root, finely chopped

¼ cup fresh celery leaves, finely chopped

1 tbsp of fresh basil, finely chopped

Salt and pepper to taste

5 tbsp extra virgin olive oil

Preparation:

Preheat the oil in a large non-stick frying pan over a medium-high temperature. Add finely chopped celery root, celery leaves, and fresh basil. Season with salt and pepper and stir-fry for about 10 minutes, until nicely browned.

Add chopped tomatoes and about ¼ cup of water. Reduce the heat to minimum and cook for 15 minutes, stirring constantly, until softened. Now add about 4 cups of water (or vegetable broth) and bring it to a boil. Give it a good stir and remove from the heat.

Top with fresh parsley and serve.

Nutrition information per serving: Kcal: 182, Protein: 1.4g, Carbs: 6.9g, Dietary Fibers: 1.9g, Sugars: 3.5g, Fats: 17.8g, Saturated Fats: 2.6g

17. Creamy Wild Asparagus Soup

Ingredients:

2 lbs fresh wild asparagus, trimmed

2 small onions, peeled and finely chopped

1 cup of heavy cream

4 cups of vegetable broth

2 tbsp of butter

1 tbsp of vegetable oil

½ tsp of salt

½ tsp of dried oregano

½ tsp of cayenne pepper

Preparation:

Rinse and drain asparagus. Cut into about one inch thick pieces. Set aside.

Melt the butter in a large skillet and add oil. Heat up and add onions. Cook until translucent.

Now add trimmed asparagus, oregano, salt, and cayenne pepper. Stir well and continue to cook until asparagus soften.

Add the vegetable broth and mix well to combine. Cook for 15 minutes, stirring occasionally.

Whisk in one cup of heavy cream and serve.

Nutrition information per serving: Kcal: 284, Protein: 11g, Carbs: 14.1g, Dietary Fibers: 5.6g, Sugars: 6.5g, Fats: 22g, Saturated Fats: 11.7g

18.   Toasted Pine Nuts Salad

Ingredients:

2 oz of Swiss chard, chopped

1 medium-sized yellow bell pepper, sliced

1 small green apple, cored and chopped

¼ cup of pine nuts, lightly toasted

¼ of fennel bulb, chopped into bite-sized pieces

2 tbsp of coconut

½ tsp of pink Himalayan salt

½ tsp of black pepper, ground

Preparation:

Mix together vinegar, salt, and pepper in a mixing bowl. Set aside.

Combine the vegetables in a large bowl. Add apple slices and pine nuts. Toss well to combine and serve.

Nutritional information per serving: Calories: 85, Protein: 2.0g Carbs: 8.8g Fats: 5.6g

19.   Brown Rice Pudding with Raspberries and Chia Seeds

Ingredients:

¾ cup of brown rice

1 cup of almond milk

¼ cup of honey

1 tbsp of coconut oil

¼ tsp of pink Himalayan salt

½ cup of raspberries

¼ cup of walnuts

2 tbsp of chia seeds

Preparation:

Bring 2 cups of water to a boil. Add rice and reduce the heat. Cover and cook for about 15 minutes.

Now add one cup of almond milk, honey, coconut oil, and salt. Continue to cook for five more minutes. Remove from the heat and cool for a while.

Top with fresh raspberries, walnuts, and chia seeds. Serve.

Nutrition information per serving: Kcal: 451, Protein: 8.6g, Carbs: 53.9g, Fats: 24.6g

20.   Avocado Pineapple Salad

Ingredients:

1 cup of avocado chunks

1 cup of pineapple chunks

1 cup of watermelon

1 cup of sour cream

1 cup of spinach, finely chopped

1 tbsp of honey

1 tsp of vanilla extract

1 tbsp of flaxseeds

Preparation:

In a medium bowl, combine sour cream, honey, vanilla extract, and flaxseeds. Stir well to combine and set aside.

Wash and prepare the vegetables.

Peel the avocado and pineapple and cut in half. Remove the pit from the avocado and cut into small chunks along with pineapple. Place in a large salad bowl and set aside.

Cut one large watermelon wedge and peel it. Cut into bite-sized pieces and discard the seeds. Add it to the bowl with other fruits and set aside.

Wash the spinach thoroughly under cold running water and roughly chop it. Add it to the bowl with other fruits.

Now, pour the sour cream mixture over the fruits and veggies and toss well to coat all the ingredients.

Refrigerate for 15 minutes before serving.

Nutrition information per serving: Kcal: 346, Protein: 4.7g, Carbs: 25.5g, Fats: 26.5g

21.   Green Delicious Apples with Broccoli

Ingredients

2 cups of broccoli, halved

2 large green delicious apples, roughly chopped

2 tbsp of olive oil

1 tbsp of dried parsley

½ tsp of pink Himalayan salt

3 cups of water

Preparation:

Bring the water to boil in a deep pot. Add broccoli and cook for about 20 minutes, or until soft. You can try this with a fork. Remove from the heat and drain. Allow it to cool for a while and cut each broccoli in half.

Wash and roughly chop the apples. Combine it with broccoli in a bowl and season with olive oil and salad seasoning.

Nutrition information per serving: Kcal: 291 Protein: 4.2g, Carbs: 13.2g, Fats: 14.7g

22.   Almond Milk and Spinach Smoothie

Ingredients:

2 cups of baby spinach, roughly chopped

1 cup of almond milk

½ avocado, roughly chopped

½ cup fresh mint leaves

1 cup of water

1 tbsp of honey

A handful of ice cubes

Preparation:

Combine the ingredients in a blender and pulse until smoot. Serve cold.

Nutrition information per serving: Kcal: 427 Protein: 5.3g, Carbs: 22.6g, Fats: 38.7g

23.   Homemade Chicken Soup

Ingredients:

1 lb chicken meat

½ cup of soup noodles

4 cups of chicken broth

A handful of fresh parsley

1 tsp of salt

¼ tsp of freshly ground black pepper

Preparation:

For this recipe, I always try to find an organic chicken. They are much tastier and better for a homemade soup. Use both, dark and white pieces and rinse well under the running water. Pat dry with a kitchen paper and place on a clean work surface.

Using a sharp paring knife, cut chicken into bite-sized pieces. Sprinkle with salt and place in a deep pot. If using organic chicken, be careful not to add extra fat because this meat already has enough fat.

Pour in the chicken broth and cover with a lid. Cook for 45 minutes, over medium-high heat.

Now add soup noodles and reduce the heat to minimum. Cook for five more minutes.

Sprinkle with some freshly ground black pepper and parsley.

Serve warm.

Nutrition information per serving: Kcal: 282, Protein: 38.6g, Carbs: 6g, Dietary Fibers: 0g, Sugars: 0.6g, Fats: 10.2g, Saturated Fats: 2.8g

24. Swiss Chard Stew with Soft Chicken Meat

Ingredients:

2 lbs chicken meat, dark and white meat

2 lbs Swiss chard, chopped

2 cups of chicken broth

2 tbsp butter, unsalted

2 tbsp olive oil

1 tsp sea salt

Preparation:

Thoroughly rinse the meat and pat dry with a kitchen paper. Using a sharp paring knife, cut the meat into smaller pieces.

Rinse well the Swiss chard. Always look for organic vegetables. They can be a bit messier to clean but are definitely worth it. Chop and drain in a colander.

Place the meat in a large, heavy-bottomed pot. Add two cups of chicken broth, season with salt, and bring it to a boil. Cook until fork-tender. Remove from the heat and drain. Reserve the liquid for some other recipe.

In the same pot, melt the butter over medium-high heat. Add Swiss chard and stir-fry for five minutes. Season with salt, pepper, or some turmeric. Serve with chicken.

Nutrition information per serving: Kcal: 484, Protein: 57.8g, Carbs: 7.2g, Dietary Fibers: 3g, Sugars: 2.3g, Fats: 24.7g, Saturated Fats: 7.6g

25.   Kidney Bean Stew

Ingredients:

7 oz red beans, pre-cooked

2 medium-sized carrots, chopped

2 celery stalks

1 large onion, peeled and finely chopped

2 tbsp of tomato paste

1 tbsp of all-purpose flour

½ tbsp of cayenne pepper

1 bay leaf

1 cup of vegetable broth

3 tbsp of extra virgin olive oil

1 tsp of salt

A handful of fresh parsley

Preparation:

Rinse well the celery stalks and cut into about half-inch thick pieces. Set aside.

Peel the carrots to remove the outer layers. Using a sharp paring knife, finely chop each carrot into small pieces.

Heat up the olive oil in a medium-sized skillet and add onions. Sautee until translucent. Add celery stalks and chopped carrots. Continue to cook for five more minutes, adding one tablespoon of vegetable broth at the time.

Now add red beans, cayenne pepper, bay leaf, salt, parsley, and tomato paste. Stir in one tablespoon of all-purpose flour and pour in the remaining vegetable broth.

Cook for 25 minutes, over medium-high heat, stirring constantly.

Sprinkle with some fresh parsley and serve warm.

Nutrition information per serving: Kcal: 311, Protein: 13.7g, Carbs: 40.8g, Dietary Fibers: 9.8g, Sugars: 5.5g, Fats: 11.6g, Saturated Fats: 1.7g

26.   Lean Shrimp Stew with Brussels Sprouts

Ingredients:

1 lb of large shrimps, cleaned

7 oz of Brussels sprouts, outer leaves removed

5 oz of okra, whole

2 small carrots, sliced

3 oz of baby corn

2 cups of chicken broth

2 large tomatoes, diced

2 tbsp of tomato paste

½ tsp of chili pepper, ground

¼ tsp of black pepper, freshly ground

1 tsp of sea salt

1 cup of olive oil

¼ cup of balsamic vinegar

1 tbsp of fresh rosemary, finely chopped

1 small celery stalk, for decoration

2 tbsp of sour cream, optionally

Preparation:

Wash the shrimps under cold running water and drain in a large colander. Set aside.

Combine olive oil, balsamic vinegar, rosemary, salt, and pepper in a large bowl. Stir well and place the shrimps into the bowl. Toss well to coat and refrigerate for 20 minutes to allow flavors to meld into the shrimps.

Meanwhile, wash and prepare the vegetables. Trim off the outer layers of the Brussels sprouts and slice the carrots.

First, place diced tomatoes a deep pot, along with tomato paste, 2 tablespoons of olive oil, and chili pepper. Cook for 15 minutes, over medium-high heat, stirring constantly. Remove the sauce to a medium-sized bowl and cover with a lid. Set aside.

Now, pour the chicken broth into your pot and add Brussels sprouts, carrots, and okra. Sprinkle with some salt, pepper, and cover. Simmer for 20 minutes, stirring occasionally.

When the vegetables are fork-tender, remove them from the pot. Set aside.

Place the shrimps in the remaining broth and bring it to a boil. Add some water if necessary and cook for 7 minutes. Drain and set aside.

Preheat the remaining oil in a large saucepan over a medium-high heat. Add previously cooked vegetables and add baby corn. Stir well and cook for about 2-3 minutes. Remove from the heat and transfer to a serving bowl. Add shrimps and tomato sauce.

Nutrition information per serving: Kcal: 193, Protein: 15.7g, Carbs: 20g, Dietary Fibers: 4.3g, Sugars: 5.2g, Fats: 7.2g, Saturated Fats: 1.4g

27.   Leek Omelet

Ingredients:

1 lb fresh leek, chopped into bite-sized pieces

7-8 garlic cloves, whole

1 tbsp butter, unsalted

2 tbsp olive oil

4 large eggs

1 tsp salt

Preparation:

In a large skillet, heat up the olive oil and add chopped leek and whole garlic cloves. Stir-fry for ten minutes, stirring constantly.

Stir in one tablespoon of butter and add eggs but make sure to keep them whole. This recipe requires poached eggs.

Cook for 3 more minutes, and remove from the heat.

Serve immediately.

Nutrition information per serving: Kcal: 468, Protein: 16.7g, Carbs: 36.3g, Dietary Fibers: 4.3g, Sugars: 9.7g, Fats: 30.4g, Saturated Fats: 8.8g

28.　　Spring Spinach Smoothie

Ingredients:

¼ cup of spinach, finely chopped

¼ cup of broccoli, finely chopped

1 tbsp of walnuts, minced

1 tbsp of hazelnuts, minced

2 cups of water

¼ tsp of ginger, ground

A handful of ice cubes

Preparation:

Combine spinach and broccoli in a colander and wash under cold running water. Drain and place in a blender along with all other ingredients. Pulse for 30 seconds and then transfer to a serving glass.

Add some ice and serve immediately.

Nutrition information per serving: Kcal: 44, Protein: 1.7g, Carbs: 1.8g, Fats: 3.8g

29.   Lentil Burger Wraps

Ingredients:

1 cup lentils, pre-cooked

1 oz spinach, finely chopped

¼ cup feta cheese

1 tsp fresh rosemary, finely chopped

¼ cup bread crumbs

5 tbsp olive oil

1 onion, peeled and sliced

3 tbsp sweet corn

A handful of fresh lettuce, finely chopped

5-6 cherry tomatoes

5 whole grain wraps

Preparation:

In a large bowl, combine lentils with spinach, feta, rosemary, bread crumbs, and three tablespoons of olive oil. Shape bite-sized balls and gently flatten them in the middle. Set aside.

Heat up the remaining oil in a large skillet. Gently place burgers in the skillet and cook for 2-3 minutes on each side, or until light brown.

Meanwhile, sprinkle some water on each wrap and microwave for one minute. Set aside.

Divide burgers between five wraps. Add some lettuce, onions, corn, and cherry tomatoes to each wrap. Fold over and secure with some toothpicks.

Serve immediately.

Nutrition information per serving: Kcal: 496, Protein: 17.6g, Carbs: 66.6g, Dietary Fibers: 16.1g, Sugars: 5.7g, Fats: 19.5g, Saturated Fats: 3.4g

30.   Lentil Spread

Ingredients:

1 lb of lentils, pre-cooked

1 cup of sweet corn

3 large tomatoes, diced

3 tbsp of tomato paste

½ tsp of dried oregano, ground

2 tbsp of Parmesan cheese

1 tsp of salt

½ tsp of red pepper flakes

3 tbsp of olive oil

¼ cup of vegetable broth

Preparation:

Heat up some olive oil in a medium-sized pot. Add diced tomatoes, tomato paste, and ½ cup of water. Sprinkle with some oregano and bring it to a boil. Cook for five minutes, stirring constantly.

Now add lentils, sweet corn, and broth. Bring it to a boil and simmer over medium heat for 15 minutes.

Remove from the heat and cool completely. Transfer to the refrigerator and chill for at least 30 minutes before serving.

Top with grated Parmesan and enjoy.

Nutrition information per serving: Kcal: 297, Protein: 17.3g, Carbs: 41.9g, Dietary Fibers: 19g, Sugars: 4.4g, Fats: 7g, Saturated Fats: 1.4g

31.   Brown Rice with Stewed Vegetables

Ingredients:

1 cup of brown rice, uncooked

8oz fresh cauliflower

2 medium-sized carrots, sliced

1 medium sized cellery root, sliced

1 tsp of pink Himalayan salt

½ tsp of freshly ground black pepper

2 tbsp of extra coconut oil

1 tablespoon of fresh celery, finely chopped

Preparation:

Place one cup of brown rice in a deep pot. Add three cups of water and bring it to a boil. Reduce the heat and continue to cook until the liquid evaporates. Remove from the heat and set aside.

Meanwhile, boil the vegetables and cook until soft. Remove from the heat and drain.

Melt the coconut oil over a medium-hogh heat. Add cooked rice, salt, pepper and stir-fry for 3-4 minutes. Mix well and serve with sliced vegetables.

Add some chopped celery and serve warm.

Nutrition information per serving: Kcal: 399 Protein: 10g, Carbs: 84.8g, Fats: 2.7g

32.   Lean Broccoli Stew with Thyme

Ingredients:

2 oz fresh broccoli

A handful of fresh parsley, finely chopped

1 tsp of dried thyme, ground

1 tbsp of freshly squeezed lemon juice

3 tbsp of coconut oil

1 tbsp of cashew cream

Preparation:

Place the broccoli in a deep pot and pour enough water to cover. Bring it to a boil and cook until tender. Remove from the heat and drain.

Transfer to a food processor. Add fresh parsley, thyme, and about ½ cup of water. Pulse until smooth mixture. Return to a pot and add some more water. Bring it to a boil and cook for several minutes, over a minimum temperature.

Stir in some coconut oil and cashew cream, sprinkle with fresh lemon juice. Serve warm.

Nutrition information per serving: Kcal: 377 Protein: 1.8g, Carbs: 4.7g, Fats: 41.2g

33.   Marinated Smelt Risotto

Ingredients:

1 lb fresh smelts, cleaned and heads removed

1 cup extra virgin olive oil

½ cup freshly squeezed lemon juice

¼ cup freshly squeezed orange juice

1 tbsp Dijon mustard

1 tsp fresh rosemary, finely chopped

2 garlic cloves, crushed

1 tsp sea salt

½ cup of rice

7 oz okra

1 large carrot, sliced

¼ cup green peas, soaked overnight

7 oz cherry tomatoes, halved

4 tbsp vegetable oil

2 cups fish stock

Preparation:

In a large bowl, combine olive oil with lemon juice, orange juice, dijon, garlic, salt, and rosemary. Stir well and submerge fish in this mixture. Refrigerate for one hour.

Meanwhile, grease the bottom of a medium-sized pot with vegetable poil. Add sliced carrots, peas, cherry tomatoes, and okra. Simmer for ten minuts, stirring constantly.

Now add rice and fish stock. Bring it to a boil and cook for ten minutes over medium-high heat.

Remove the fish from the refrigerator and add to the pot along with half of the marinade. Continue to cook for 5 more minutes.

Nutrition information per serving: Kcal: 583, Protein: 30.1g, Carbs: 24.7g, Dietary Fibers: 3.2g, Sugars: 4.4g, Fats: 40.7g, Saturated Fats: 6.8g

34.   Citrus Catfish Fillets

Ingredients:

1 lb catfish fillets

1 cup of olive oil

½ lemon, sliced

¼ cup of lemon juice, freshly squeezed

1 tsp of dry rosemary, ground

1 tbsp of fresh parsley, finely chopped

3 garlic cloves, crushed

¼ tsp of pink Himalayan salt

Preparation:

Rinse the fillets under cold running water and pat dry with a kitchen paper.

Combine the olive oil, lemon juice, rosemary, parsley, garlic, and salt in a bowl and stir well. Submerge the fillets in this mixture and refrigerate for 30 minutes (it can stand in the refrigerator up to 2 hours).

Meanwhile, preheat the oven to 300 degrees. Line some parchment paper over a baking sheet and set aside.

Remove the fish from the refrigerator and transfer to a baking sheet. Add half of the marinade and cook for about 30 minutes.

Remove from the oven, sprinkle with some more marinade and serve with lemon slices and some vegetables of your choice.

Nutrition information per serving: Kcal: 421, Protein: 27g, Carbs: 2.6g, Fats: 34g

35.   Roasted Pecans and Arugula Salad

Ingredients:

1 lb of fresh arugula, chopped

1 large apple, pitted and wedged

2 tbsp of lemon juice, freshly squeezed

1 small onion, sliced

2 tbsp of extra-virgin olive oil

2 oz of pecans, roughly chopped

1 tbsp of liquid honey

1 tsp of pink Himalayan salt

¼ tsp of black pepper, freshly ground

Preparation:

Preheat the oven to 300°F.

Line some parchment paper over a baking sheet and spread nuts over it. Place it in the oven and bake for 10 minutes, or until golden brown. Remove from the oven and set aside to cool for a while.

In a small bowl, combine lemon juice, oil, honey, salt, and pepper. Stir until well incorporated and set aside to allow flavors to meld.

Wash the arugula thoroughly under cold running water. Drain and roughly chop it in a large salad bowl. Set aside.

Wash the apple and cut in half. Remove the core and slice the apple into wedges. Add it to the bowl with arugula and set aside.

Peel the onion and slice into thin slices. Add it to the bowl with other ingredients.

Now, drizzle the salad with dressing and toss well until coat all the ingredients. Top with roasted pecans and serve immediately.

Nutrition information per serving: Kcal: 241, Protein: 4.9g, Carbs: 20.1g, Fats: 18g

36.   Rice Rolls

Ingredients:

40 wine leaves, fresh

1 cup of brown rice

2 tbsp olive oil

3 garlic cloves, crushed

¼ cup of lemon juice, freshly squeezed

2 tbsp fresh mint

½ tsp of pink Himalayan salt

Preparation:

Wash the leaves thoroughly, one at a time. Place on a clean working surface. Grease the bottom of a deep pot with oil and make a layer with wine leaves. Set aside.

In a medium-sized bowl, combine rice with oil, garlic, mint, salt, and pepper. Place one wine leaf at a time on a working surface and add one teaspoon of filling at the bottom end. Fold the leaf over the filling towards the center. Bring the two sides in towards the center and roll them up tightly. Gently transfer to a pot.

Add 2 cups of water and lemon juice. Cover and cook for 30 minutes, over medium-high heat.

Remove from the pot and chill overnight in the refrigerator.

Nutrition information per serving: Kcal: 313, Protein: 2.9g, Carbs: 30.4, Fats: 20.5g

37.   Asian Asparagus Salad

Ingredients:

1 lb of wild asparagus, trimmed

1 cup of spring onions, chopped

1 cup of red cabbage, chopped

1 tbsp of white wine vinegar

1 tbsp of olive oil

½ tsp of ginger, freshly grated

½ tsp of pink Himalayan salt

¼ tsp of black pepper, ground

Preparation:

Place the asparagus in a pot of boiling water. Cook for about 3-5 minutes, or until soften. Remove from the heat and soak in cold water for a while.

Meanwhile, combine canola oil, ginger, vinegar, chili, salt, and pepper in a mixing bowl.

Drain well the asparagus and place in a large bowl and add spring onions and red cabbage. Drizzle with dressing and toss all well to coat. Serve immediately.

Nutrition information per serving: Kcal: 91, Protein: 4.3g, Carbs: 10.2g, Fats: 5.0g

38.   Citrus Quinoa Porridge

Ingredients:

1 cup of white quinoa

2 tbsp of lemon juice, freshly squeezed

¼ tsp of pink Himalayan salt

1 tsp of lemon zest, freshly grated

2 cups of vegetable stock, unsalted

1 tbsp of coconut oil

Preparation:

Combine quinoa and water in a medium pot. Bring it to a boil and then reduce the heat to low. Add lemon juice and butter. Sprinkle with lemon zest and a pinch of salt. Cover with a lid and cook for another 15 minutes. Remove from the heat and serve.

Nutrition information per serving: Kcal: 132, Protein: 3.7g, Carbs: 18.1g, Fats: 6.8g

39.   Red Pollock Stew

Ingredients:

1 lb pollock fillet

4 garlic cloves, crushed

4 large tomatoes, peeled

2 bay leaves, whole

2 cups fish stock

1 teaspoon freshly ground black pepper

1 large onion, peeled and finely chopped

½ cup extra virgin olive oil

1 teaspoon sea salt

Preparation:

In a large skillet, heat up two tablespoons of olive oil. Add finely chopped onion and cook until translucent, stirring constantly. Add tomatoes and continue to cook until completely soft, adding some fish stock from time to time.

When tomatoes have softened and the liquid has evaporated, add the remaining ingredients and one cup of water. Bring it to a boil and cook for 15 minutes.

Nutrition information per serving: Kcal: 404, Protein: 28.1g, Carbs: 9.5g, Dietary Fibers: 2.6g, Sugars: 5.1g, Fats: 28.9g, Saturated Fats: 4.5g

40.   Sesame Seed Risotto with Lamb

Ingredients:

1 cup of rice

1 cup of green peas

14 oz of lamb, tender cuts

3 tbsp of sesame seeds

3 cups of beef broth

1 tsp of sea salt

1 bay leaf

½ tsp of dried thyme

3 tbsp of butter

Preparation:

Wash the meat and place on a clean working surface. Slice into approximately 1/2-inch thick slices. Place in the pressure cooker and add beef broth. Close the lid and set the steam release handle. Cook for about 20 minutes, depending on thype of your cooker. Release the steam and remove the meat, but reserve the liquid. The meat should be fork-tender.

Transfer to a deep pot. Add rice, green peas, and the remaining broth. Bring it to a boil and reduce the heat to minimum. Simmer for 10 more minutes, stirring occasionally.

Remove from the heat and stir in three tablespoons of butter and sesame seeds.

Serve immediately.

Nutrition information per serving: Kcal: 498, Protein: 34.4g, Carbs: 43.9g, Dietary Fibers: 3.3g, Sugars: 2.1g, Fats: 19.7g, Saturated Fats: 8.6g

41.   Spinach and Lamb Soup

Ingredients:

1 lb lamb rack

7 oz spinach, torn

2 medium-sized onions, finely chopped

3 tbsp olive oil

4 cups beef broth

½ tsp sea salt

½ tsp Italian seasoning mix

Preparation:

Rinse well the meat and rub with sea salt and Italian seasoning mix. Place in a deep pot and add broth. Bring it to a boil and cook for 45 minutes.

Remove from the heat and set aside.

Grease the bottom of a large skillet with olive oil. Add onions and stir-fry for 5 minutes. Now add spinach and continue to cook for 5 more minutes.

Finally, add meat, broth, and one more cup of water. Bring it to a boil and remove from the heat.

Serve immediately.

Nutrition information per serving: Kcal: 373, Protein: 38.7g, Carbs: 7.8g, Dietary Fibers: 2.3g, Sugars: 3.2g, Fats: 20.4g, Saturated Fats: 4.9g

42.   Beet Apple and Spinach Salad

Ingredients:

1 large beet, steamed and sliced

2 cups of spinach, trimmed

2 spring onions, finely chopped

1 small green apple

¼ cup of olive oil

2 tbsp of fresh lime juice

1 tbsp of honey

1 garlic clove, crushed

1 tsp of apple cider

¼ tsp of freshly ground black pepper

¼ tsp of pink Himalayan salt

Preparation:

Place the beet in a deep pot. Pour enough water to cover and cook for about 40 minutes, or until tender. Remove the skin and slice. Transfer to a bowl. Combine olive oil, vinegar, cider, salt, pepper, and honey. Pour over beet slices and toss to coat. Let it stand for at least 30 minutes.

Wash and pat dry the apple. Slice into thin strips and combine with beet slices, spring onions, and spinach. Add crushed garlic and mix well. Serve.

Nutrition information per serving: Kcal: 365 Protein: 3.3g, Carbs: 37.1g, Fats: 25.8g

43.   Beet Greens and Kale with Garlic Dressing

Ingredients:

1 cup of beet greens, rinsed and chopped

2 cups of kale, rinsed and chopped

2 spring onions, finely chopped

For dressing:

2 garlic cloves, crushed

3 tbsp of cilantro, finely chopped

1 orange

¼ cup of raw cashews

¼ cup of olive oil

A pinch of pink Himalayan salt

Preparation:

Combine the dressing ingredients in a food processor and mix well until creamy mixture. Set aside.

Place the beet greens in a sauce pan and pour enough water to cover. Bring it to a boil and cook for a couple of minutes. Remove from the heat and drain. Cool for a while and transfer to a bowl. Add chopped kale and spring onion, pour the dressing over the salad and toss well to combine.

Nutrition information per serving: Kcal: 407 Protein: 6.8g, Carbs: 26.6g, Fats: 33.4g

44.   Thick Fish Soup with Peas

Ingredients:

7 oz mackerel fillets

½ cup wheat groats, soaked

½ cup kidney beans, soaked

¼ cup sweet corn

1 lb fresh tomatoes, peeled and roughly chopped

4 cups fish stock

4 tbsp extra virgin olive oil

1 tsp sea salt

1 tsp fresh rosemary, finely chopped

3 garlic cloves, crushed

Preparation:

Grease the botton of a deep pot with olive oil. Add crushed garlic and tomatoes and cook for 5 minutes over medium heat.

Now add rosemary, fish stock, salt, corn, kidney beans, and wheat groats. Cover and reduce the heat to minimum. Simmer for 20 minutes.

Finally, add mackerel fillets and cook for 10 more minutes.

Serve immediately.

Nutrition information per serving: Kcal: 479, Protein: 26.8g, Carbs: 38.3g, Dietary Fibers: 8.2g, Sugars: 3.9g, Fats: 25.7g, Saturated Fats: 4.7g

45.   Thick Lentil Soup

Ingredients:

1 cup of brown lentils

1 large onion, peeled and finely chopped

2 large carrots, sliced

1 large sweet potato, peeled and chopped

2 large celery stalks, sliced

3 tbsp of extra virgin olive oil

3 large garlic cloves, minced

4 cups of beef broth

1 tsp of thyme, dried

1 tsp of salt

¼ tsp of freshly ground black pepper

Preparation:

In a medium-sized pot, heat up the oil and add onions, garlic, and sliced celery. Cook for 5 minutes, stirring constantly.

Now add lentils, sliced carrot, and chopped potato. Stir in salt, pepper, and thyme. Pour in the broth and stir well.

Cover with the lid and bring it to a boil. Reduce the heat to minimum and simmer for 20 minutes.

Remove from the heat and serve immediately.

Nutrition information per serving: Kcal: 541, Protein: 30.8g, Carbs: 44.3g, Dietary Fibers: 14.9g, Sugars: 4.7g, Fats: 26.7g, Saturated Fats: 7g

46.   Egg Salad

Ingredients:

3 eggs, boiled

1 yellow bell pepper, sliced and seeds removed

1 red onion, sliced

1 medium-sized tomato, roughly chopped

1 small cucumber, sliced

a handful of lettuce, torn

7 oz fresh goat's cheese

1 tsp sea salt

4 tbsp extra virgin olive oil

1 tbsp freshly squeezed lemon juice

Preparation:

Boil a medium-sized pot of water. Gently place the eggs in it and cook for 10 minutes. Remove from the heat and drain. Cool for a while.

Meanwhile, combine vegetables in a large bowl. Peel and slice eggs. Transfer to a bowl. Add fresh goat's cheese and season with salt.

Drizzle with olive oil and freshly squeezed lemon juice. Serve immediately.

Nutrition information per serving: Kcal: 389, Protein: 16.4g, Carbs: 11.1g, Fats: 32.4g

ADDITIONAL TITLES FROM THIS AUTHOR

70 Effective Meal Recipes to Prevent and Solve Being Overweight: Burn Fat Fast by Using Proper Dieting and Smart Nutrition

By Joe Correa CSN

48 Acne Solving Meal Recipes: The Fast and Natural Path to Fixing Your Acne Problems in Less Than 10 Days!

By Joe Correa CSN

41 Alzheimer's Preventing Meal Recipes: Reduce or Eliminate Your Alzheimer's Condition in 30 Days or Less!

By Joe Correa CSN

70 Effective Breast Cancer Meal Recipes: Prevent and Fight Breast Cancer with Smart Nutrition and Powerful Foods

By Joe Correa CSN

www.ingramcontent.com/pod-product-compliance
Lightning Source LLC
Chambersburg PA
CBHW051033030426
42336CB00015B/2845